JESUS STILL HEALS TODAY

Mark 10:27

By Dr Liya Mutale

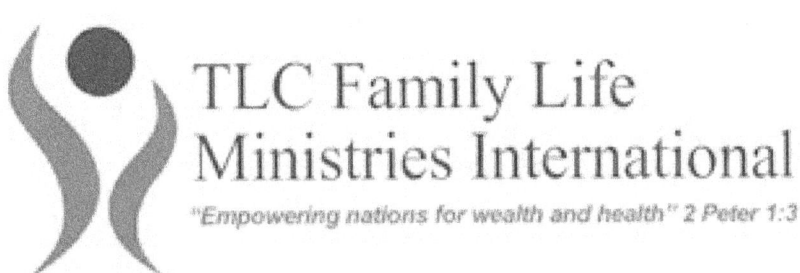

TLC Family Life
Ministries International

"Empowering nations for wealth and health" 2 Peter 1:3

Tender Loving Care (TLC) Family Life Ministries International offers teaching sessions on important Family Life issues to "Empower Nations for Wealth and Health". TLC believes that God has given us everything we need in a seed, and therefore TLC endeavor to help you grow that seed to its full potential. **2 Peter 1:3.**
For more information **email us on tflmibooks@yahoo.com**

ACKNOWLEDGEMENTS

First and foremost I would like to give God the glory and the honor for giving me the wisdom and the strength to write another book. I want to acknowledge and thank my family for the support and love that they have shown me even in my times of sickness. I write this book fully convinced that Jesus still heals today. I also thank and acknowledge the Men and Women of God whom God used to inspire me to write this book. A special thank you goes to my husband Brig. Gen. Justin Mutale for helping me edit the book and for the encouragement he gave me to write it.

I also want to thank my friend and sister in the Lord, Dr Sampa Chitambala Otiono for introducing me to the Healthcare Christian Fellowship for which I hope this book will be a useful resource as the healthcare workers minister salvation and divine healing to their patients throughout Zambia and beyond. My prayer now is that may the intended purpose of writing this book, which is to minister divine healing to those in need of healing in the body, be fulfilled. Be blessed, healed, and delivered in Jesus name, Amen.

TABLE OF CONTENTS

CHAPTER ONE

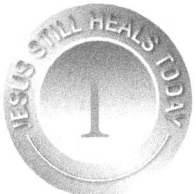

HEALING IS GOD'S WILL FOR YOU

The truth of the matter is that God wants His children well. If you are a child of God and not only His creation, you must know that God wants you completely whole, spirit, soul and body. God has good plans for us, plans to prosper us, and plans to give us a hope and a future. (Jeremiah 29:11)

God made His intentions very clear when He sent is begotten son Jesus to die on the cross for our healing and salvation. When we accept the Lord Jesus Christ as our Lord and savior we receive the gift of righteousness which puts us in right standing with God. From this position of righteousness we are given authority and dominion over the earth and everything in it. Therefore in this position of righteousness we can create at a command because of the power that Jesus Christ left us with through the Holy Spirit.

If God could have loved us so much as to let His only begotten son Jesus Christ die on the Cross of Calvary, how then would He not want us healed. Jesus Christ at the Cross cried out "it is finished", and indeed every sickness, disease, curse and poverty was taken away. In 1 Peter 2:24 the Bible tells us that, "He himself bore our sins on his body on the cross, so that we might die to sin and live for righteousness; by his wounds you have been healed". So it is very clear here that we were healed when Jesus went to the cross to die for us, but nevertheless, Jesus demonstrated his desire to heal during his earthly ministry long before he went to die on the Cross. In the book of Acts Chapter 10:38 the Bible records, "How God anointed Jesus of Nazareth with the Holy Spirit and Power, and he went around doing good and healing all who were under the power of the devil, because God was with him". With this anointing, Mathew 4:23 says, "Jesus went throughout Galilee, teaching in their Synagogues, preaching the good news of the Kingdom and healing every disease and sickness among the people".

In the Old Testament, we see that God's used the Law to promise healing to the children of Israel, so it was dependent on whether or not they were obedient to the Lord our God. Most of the healing promises made in the Old Testament came with a condition, so that if the children of Israel obeyed then healing came. Let us look at a few scriptures; in Exodus 23:25 -26; "Worship the Lord your God, and his blessing will be on your food and water. I will take away sickness from among you, and none will miscarry or be barren in your land. I will give you a full life span". Proverbs 4:20-22; "My son, attend to my words, incline thine ear unto my sayings. Let them not depart from thine eyes; keep them in the midst of thine heart. For they are life unto those that find them, and health to all their flesh".

In the New Testament, God's Laws are written in our hearts and in order to receive our healing God requires us to have FAITH. It is the faith that we have in the fact that Jesus took our sicknesses and infirmities on the Cross that brings healing. The Bible clearly tells us that, EVERYTHING IS POSSIBILE to them that believe. So if you believe that Jesus took your sickness away, then your healing will manifest itself. You are healed according to your faith.

CHAPTER TWO

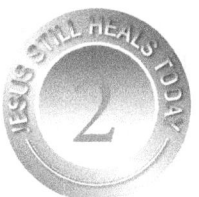

SOME SPIRITUAL ROOT CAUSES OF DISEASE

What we need to understand is that as human beings we are a triune being with a spirit, soul and body. When one of these has a problem it affects the other two parts. It is important to understand this as we begin to look at the spiritual root causes of disease.

SIN

Sin can be an open door for sickness and disease. So many Christians and non-Christians alike have through sin opened spiritual doors that are causing havoc in their lives. Every time we sin we open a spiritual door that allows the enemy to come in and destroy our lives. We should first accept the Lord Jesus Christ as our Lord and savior, repent of our sins and pursue a holy life without sin. After which we need to command all evil spirits that came in through those open doors to leave us in Jesus name and sin no more. Jesus told the people he healed to go and sin no more.

Before you begin to pray for healing, it is important that you do an introspection of your life. Sin, such as disobedience, rebellion, bitterness, anger, unforgiveness, sexual sin, addiction, alcoholism etc can open doors for the devil to cause sickness. The devil only comes to steal, kill and destroy. The devil will not harm you if you do not have anything that belongs to him, but if you have sin the devil will have permission to disturb your life including bringing sickness to your body.

In order to resist the devil in this case we need to try as much as possible to walk in holiness. God asks as to be holy as He is holy; therefore I want to assume that it is very possible to live a sin free life. Sin such as bitterness and unforgiveness usually causes diseases such as hypertension, cancer, chest infections and throat infections. While practicing medicine in the Lusaka Urban Clinics I saw many patients recover and get healed after they decided to let go of anger or after they chose to forgive. The idea that bitterness and unforgiveness were a source of many health problems never made sense to me in the earlier years of my practice, but over time I became convinced that one of the greatest thieves of happiness, joy and good health is the unwillingness to let go of hurtful incidences in one's life. It is also important to realize that at least over 50% of the physical elements we suffer from are caused by disturbances in our 'soul' such as anger, bitterness, and unforgiveness.

REPENTANCE PREPARES THE WAY TO HEALING

Repentance is the first step to healing and restoration. Repentance means to turn from ones sins and dedicate oneself to the amendment of one's life: to change one's mind. Because sin will usually take us away from the presence of God, it is important to ask forgiveness from God and quickly restore your relationship to God. Once you have restored your relationship to God it is also important to restore your relationship with the people who could have caused you to sin. True repentance will restore you to fellowship with God and with man. Unforgiveness will eat you up and not the person you are angry with. In some cases you would need to also forgive yourself and stop condemning yourself.

No matter what you have done, true repentance prepares the way for God to move in your life. The Bible tells us that without holiness we will not see God. If you have noticed in your own life, it is very difficult to hear God and receive instruction when you have sin that you have not repented of. 1 John 1:9 reads, "If we confess our sins, he is faithful and just and will forgive us our sins and purify us from all unrighteousness". Repent and come clean with God. This will prepare the way for the Lord to move in every area of your life including divine healing.

STRESS

Stress is also a common cause of sickness and diseases such as ulcers, irritable bowel, Crohn's disease, heart attacks, strokes, high blood pressure, diabetes, insomnia and so on. Research shows that 75% of visits to the doctor's office are stress-related. Stress is really almost unavoidable but establishing the reason for the stress and dealing with it would probably yield more results than prayer alone.

Other emotional disturbances such as the feeling of rejection, self-condemnation, betrayal, fear, guilt, grief and loss can equally cause disease. Anything that disturbs our emotions has the potential to cause sickness in the body. The body will normally just respond to what is happening in our soul. Therefore it is imperative that we remain stress free by learning to trust God more in any circumstances we find ourselves in.

SPIRITUAL FOUNDATIONS

I will not dwell much on these, but I think it is important for me to mention them and it will be important for you to look at these issues at individual level. Some sicknesses and diseases may be caused by evil spiritual foundations in our lives. Physically when we say 'foundation' we are refereeing to a physical structure made of concrete, iron rods and gravel. This foundation is what holds the building upright.

Spiritually, the foundation refers to the early beginnings of a life as laid by our parents and ancestors. It refers to the very first thing to which our spiritual lives have been anchored. These foundations whether spiritual or physical can be faulty and if not taken care of, can lead to destruction. A life built on a faulty foundation can bring forth bad fruit that includes sickness and disease. So it is important to find out about your foundation, the circumstances under which you were born, what your names mean and what words were spoken at your birth. After you find out these details you can renounce the evil foundations, pray for spiritual repair and declare a new foundation in Jesus name.

THE SINS OF OUR FOREFATHERS AND OUR BLOODLINES

These are known as iniquities. The consequences of the sins of our forefathers can to some extent affect our lives. Because we are connected to our forefathers and ancestors through our bloodline, we also tend to suffer the consequences of their sin. It is well known that our forefathers worshiped idols and took part in many spiritual rituals that affect our lives today. Whenever you discover strange occurrences in your life and in your family in spite of all your efforts to walk in holiness, you must look beyond the physical and examine your bloodline. Whether we know it or not the spiritual powers of our bloodline continue to have influence on our lives and destiny.

The Bible in Genesis 49:5-7 says, "Simeon and Levi are brothers – their swords are weapons of violence. Let me not enter their council, let me not join their assembly, for they have killed men in their anger and hamstrung oxen as they pleased. Cursed be their anger, so fierce, and fury, so cruel! I will scatter them in Jacob and disperse them in Israel". Here we discover that cruelty and anger were in the bloodline of Simeon and Levi. In Exodus 2:1-2 we see that a man went out of the house of Levi and took to wife a daughter of Levi and she conceived and bore a son who was Moses. So here we see that one from the bloodline of cruelty and anger married a woman who also was in the bloodline of cruelty and anger and bore a son, Moses.

Moses grew up in Pharaohs palace, enjoyed the best education and he was a prince of Egypt. He was called by God to deliver the children of Israel out of Egypt; He spoke to God face to face. But despite all this Moses killed an Egyptian in anger. The cruelty and anger of his forefathers followed him. Coming down Mount Sinai, when he saw the people worshiping idols, his anger waxed hot and he threw the stone tablets that God wrote on with His own fingers. His anger was strong enough to hinder him from entering the Promised Land. The evil powers of his forefathers ensured that he did not reach his destiny. From this we see that even if Moses was close to God, the sins of his forefathers followed him and caused confusion in his life. Unless you deal with these strongholds by addressing them and disconnecting yourself from the evil bloodline they will be forever in your way. Eventually we also see that when Moses died the devil came to contest for his corpse. He said: "This is one of us; he has the spirit of anger. He is a murderer."

Let us take a look at another portion of scripture. In Judges 6:25, "That same night the Lord said to him (Gideon), 'Take the second bull from your father's herd, the one seven years old. Tear down your father's altar to Baal and cut down the Asherah pole beside it. Then build a proper kind of altar to the Lord your God on top of this height. Using the wood of the Asherah pole that you cut down, offer the second bull as a burnt offering".

Gideon was called by God to deliver His people as a mighty man of valor. But Gideon was only able to rise into his calling after he had dealt with the altars of his father which were affecting him negatively. Unfortunately many of us are still being controlled by the idols and evil spiritual altars of our fathers and forefathers. We need to break loose by the blood of Jesus Christ so that we can move on in our lives. So sometimes the answer to your sickness or infirmity may be a prayer cutting you free from your evil ancestral bloodline.

CHAPTER THREE

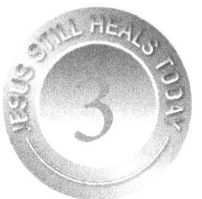

HE HEALS ALL DISEASES

So many have died and still continue to die from so called incurable diseases like Diabetes, Hypertension, Cancer and HIV/AIDS, both Christians and non-Christians alike. The fact is that you could have diabetes, hypertension, cancer or HIV but the truth is you were healed when Jesus said, "It is finished". These are all diseases like any other in the eyes of God.

It is amazing how so many Pastors do not have faith that a person infected by HIV or any other so called "incurable" disease can be healed, and yet when God talks about healing us He talks of healing all our diseases, He does not differentiate them or classify them as curable or incurable *Matt.4:23,24; Ish.53:5; Matt.8:16,17*. With God all things are possible *LK 1:37*. Jesus is the same yesterday, today and forevermore, He changeth not, *Heb. 13:8 and Matt.3:6*. There is nothing too difficult for God. *Jerm.32:27, Ps34:19, Ps 103:3*.

We need to renew our minds to believe that God can heal even HIV/AIDS, we need to prevent ourselves from listening and dwelling on the messages we hear on TV and radio about HIV/AIDS. The devil enters your mind first and convinces your mind through your thoughts that you are positive and that you will die because there is no cure. You begin to meditate on this and eventually what you feared most happens to you, you are found to be positive.

Have you ever watched a food advert on TV and suddenly felt hungry? Have you heard someone cough and suddenly you have a need to clear your throat? We naturally move to whatever we focus our attention on. The more you think about something the stronger it takes hold of you and the more you attract it to yourself. When you watch too many of these HIV/AIDS messages, you begin to entertain the idea of being positive and eventually it really manifests itself as such.

What you need to do next is to begin to think and meditate on how great God is and who you are in Christ, think of the price Christ paid on the cross. He said it was finished when He died on the cross, remember we are partakers of the divine nature of God *(2 Peter 1:3,4),* and if we are, how can a virus control us. The virus has no power over you child of God. Whatever God did not put in you when you were created can be removed by the Word of God. We need to believe the Word of God and have faith in what the Word says, many times we would rather believe the doctor because of the effort we need to believe God, to believe what we do not see, "truth". Diseases are spirit or even just a thought that can be cast out, you have the authority to cast out devils so speak to it, remember your body is the temple of the Holy Ghost there is no room for foul spirits.

We need to seriously learn how to differentiate between the "truth" and fact. The fact could be that you are HIV positive, but the TRUTH is that you were healed by the stripes of Jesus and that you will live and not die to declare the works of the Lord. Greater is He who is within you than he who is in the world. God is not man that He should lie nor is He the son of man that He should change His mind....*Numbers 23:19.* He sent His word and healed our diseases, *Psalm 107:20.* When you have decided to believe God for your healing you cannot afford to be double minded about it. The bible says, "A double minded man is unstable in all his ways".

James 1:6-8 (KJV)

You may think that your sickness or disease is the end and that it is too overpowering for you to bear, and that God can't heal you because the world said the disease is incurable, but that is a lie from the pit of hell. God has promised never to allow more on you than he puts within you to handle, see *1 Corinthians 10:13*. He will not permit any temptation that you cannot overcome. However you must do your part too by practicing four biblical keys to defeating disease.

CHAPTER FOUR

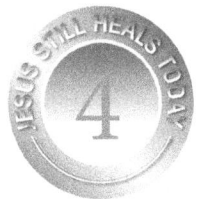

FOUR KEYS TO DEFEATING DISEASE

1. REFOCUS YOUR ATTENTION

Whatever appears on your body is a result of your mental state. You need to realize that your Spirit, Soul and Body are one and are inter-connected such that one affects the other. The spirit man in this case is constant and the body usually just manifests what the soul and the spirit have agreed on, so it is really the mind that is in play here. Fill your mind therefore with good thoughts, thoughts of peace, harmony and divine order. According to your belief it is done for you.

If you look carefully there is nowhere in the bible were we are told to *"resist temptation"* or *"resist trials"*, we are told to *"resist the devil"* (James 4:7). The thought of sickness that is in your mind is the devil you need to resist. Because most of what happens to us starts in our thoughts, the battle is basically in the mind. Now instead of trying to fight a particular thought we should resist it by refocusing our attention because fighting a thought does not work. Every time you try to block a thought out of your mind, you drive it deeper into your memory and subconscious.

The more you think about the sickness or disease and the more you try to fight the thought the more it consumes and controls you. The minute you start thinking of the disease and all that is said about it, you strengthen it. The secret is don't fight the thought, just **change** the channel of your mind and get interested in another idea. The battle is won or lost in the **MIND**. Whatever gets your attention will get to you. That is why Job in *Job 31:1* said, *"I made a covenant with my eyes not to look with lust upon a young woman"* and David prayed, *in Ps 119:37a "Keep me from paying attention to what is worthless."* You can make a covenant with your eyes and your ears not to see or hear anything that will bring fear of disease.

Sometimes I personally think you are better off not knowing too many details about diseases, the less detail you know the better for you. Sometimes people develop symptoms of a disease just because someone described to them what the symptoms are; for instance I decide to tell you that going to the bathroom frequently at night is one of the symptoms for diabetes. Suddenly because one night you go to the bathroom more than once, you decide in your mind that you have diabetes, you dwell on it, you go everywhere for a check up until you are told you have diabetes.

Ignoring the temptation to think about sickness and the fear that you will die of one disease or another is far more effective than fighting it. Once your mind moves to thinking of something else, the fear will lose its power. So when the fear of disease calls you on the phone, do not argue with it, just hang up. Sometimes this means physically leaving a place that brings these thoughts and fears, like turning off the TV, the radio or walking away from a group discussing the said consequences or symptoms of a disease. Your mind is your most vulnerable organ so to reduce the fear of disease, keep your mind occupied with God's Word and other good thoughts.

You defeat bad thoughts generally by thinking of something better. Your thought is action and the reaction is the automatic response of your body to your thoughts. Watch your thoughts! Keep your conscious mind busy with the expectation of the best, and your subconscious will faithfully reproduce your habitual thinking. This is the principle of replacement and the law of attraction. You overcome evil with good *(Romans 12:21)*. The devil can not get your attention if your mind is preoccupied with something else. That is why the bible repeatedly tells us to keep our minds focused: *"Fix your thoughts on Jesus."(Heb 3:1) "Always think about Jesus Christ." (2 Tim 2:8) "Fill your mind with those things that are good and deserve praise: things that are true, noble, right, pure, lovely and honorable."(Philip 4:8) "Be careful how you think; your life is shaped by your thoughts."* (Pro 4:23) Follow Paul's model *(2 Corin 10:5): "We capture every thought and make it give up and obey Christ."* This renewing of the mind takes a life time of practice and hard work, but with the help of the Holy Spirit you can reprogram the way you think.

The human mind and body are one and the same, different aspects of the same whole you. Unhappy thoughts are invariably reflected as disease of the body. But happy thoughts encourage a healthy body. That is a basic law.

Think about the following:

- Thought-diseases are illnesses caused or worsened by the unhappy thoughts that fill our heads.

- If you think you are sick, you are. What you think about, you bring about.

- Patients don't know that every negative thought they entertain is as dangerous as a physical germ.

- Thoughts change body chemistry.

- The best medicine is not in a bottle – it is in your head.

- A change in mental attitude often aids in the development of body resistance against disease.

2. A PROBLEM SHARED, IS A PROBLEM HALF SOLVED

You do not have to broadcast to the whole world, but you need at least one person you can honestly share your struggles with. The bible says,*(Ecc 4:9-10)* *"You are better off to have a friend than to be all alone….If you fall, your friend can help you up. But if you fall without having a friend nearby, you are really in trouble."* Some trials are only overcome with the help of a partner who prays for you, encourages you, and holds you accountable. God's plan for your growth and deliverance includes all Christians. Authentic honest fellowship is the antidote to your lonely struggle against disease. God says it is the only way you are going to break free: *(James 5:16)* *"Confess your sins to each other and pray for each other so that you may be healed."*

Do you really want to be healed? God's solution is plain: Don't repress it; confess it! Don't conceal it; reveal it. Revealing your condition is the beginning of your healing. Hiding your status only intensifies the symptoms. The situation will grow in the dark and become bigger and bigger, but when you expose it to the light of truth, it will shrink. You are only as sick as your secrets. So take off your mask, stop pretending you are perfect, and walk into freedom. This is a tool the devil has been using especially in the area of HIV; he stigmatizes people and makes them feel ashamed to reveal their status to one another, even to their Pastors.

Therefore the devil uses stigma and discrimination to threaten those who want to reveal their status to others. The devil wants you to think your positive status is unique and embarrassing so you should keep it to yourself as a secret. The truth is millions have felt what you are feeling and have faced the same struggles you're facing right now. The reason we hide our status is pride. We want others to think that we have everything "under control". **The truth is, whatever you cannot talk about is already out of control in your life**. Whenever someone confides in another, I know that they are about to experience their deliverance and healing in that area.

Yes it is humbling to admit our fears to others, but lack of humility is the very thing that is keeping you from getting better. When you are able to talk about something to another person it shows you that God is doing something about it, it means you have reach a stage where you are saying, it does not matter what anyone says I will speak out anyway. The bible says, *(James 4:6-7a)" God sets himself against the proud, but he shows favor to the humble. So humble yourselves before God."* When you go before God through a godly partner or friend to reveal your status you are humbly saying to God that you can't do it yourself, you need help. Am sure most of us have had this experience where when you decide to talk about an issue somehow it becomes lighter.

Prayer basically is us saying to God I surrender, I can't do this and then God takes over. We need to be honest in our prayers after all God is omniscient, He knows everything, so why not say it out to Him in prayer? Your prayer should be from the heart, after all God knows everything so you can't lie to Him. While you pray ensure that you have a positive mind set; if you have doubts or fear in your mind your prayer will not be answered. You don't have to impress Him with your long impressive prayers. Pray the Word of God back to Him, He is always watching to perform His Word and also remember that if you are harboring unforgiveness or sin, your prayer will not be heard, that is why it is important to confess your sins before you go into serious prayer.

Prayer is a sign of humility before God; you are saying God I can't do this I need you to help. There is a difference between God simply doing something, and doing it in the context of prayer. Doing it when we have asked for it makes it part of our relationship with Him. When I pray for something and it happens I am able to give God the Glory. I believe it is for reasons like this that God often will put the desire to pray for something in us knowing that He has already provided an answer. In fact prayer starts with God and is indeed a great privilege; it allows us to be part of God's work.

The Bible says, *"Before they call, I will answer"* (Isaiah 65:24). Indeed He answers before we call, because He puts the desire in our hearts for something He has already provided. If we listen to God before we pray we will be assured of an answer, remember God sends His word and sees to it that it is performed, His Word does not return to Him void; it accomplishes that for which He sends it. Prayer changes us not God!

3. **RESIST THE DEVIL**

After we have humbled ourselves and submitted to God in prayer, we are then told to resist the devil. The rest of James 4:7 says, *"Resist the devil and he will flee from you"*. We are not to fight back. How can we resist the devil? Paul tells us, *(Eph 6:17) "Put on salvation as your helmet, and take the sword of the Spirit, which is the Word of God."* We can resist the devil by staying away from sin. The devil is at liberty to afflict us when we are in sin because he only comes after what is his. So if you are carrying around some sin, he will come for it. The sin grants him permission to touch you.

THROUGH SALVATION

The **first step** is to accept God's salvation through the Gospel of Jesus Christ. You will not be able to say no to the devil unless you have said yes to Christ! Without Christ we are defenseless against the devil, but with the "helmet of salvation" our minds are protected by God. Remember this: If you are a believer, the devil cannot force you to do anything. He can only suggest. The Gospel of Christ is all about change. We are transformed from sinfulness to righteousness and eventually to holiness. At Calvary His poverty made us rich, by His stripes we received healing, He brought us out of the curse of the law and the chastisement of our peace was laid upon Him. As born again believers we need to be full beneficiaries of the death and resurrection of Jesus Christ, Christ came to reconnect us to

God after Adam disconnected us from him. We are Spirit beings in human bodies with the creative capabilities of God. The wisdom of God is our heritage and we are administering the affairs of this world with Christ. If we do not get the full benefits of what happened at the Cross, then Jesus suffered and died in vain.

Our reality should be that, we sit together with Christ in heavenly places; we are translated from earthly beings to heavenly beings. We have heavenly immunity as Ambassadors of Christ on earth. Because of our diplomatic immunity we cannot be harassed or mishandled by the enemy any how unless we allow it through our own thoughts and disobedience. Being born again we are translated from natural to supernatural.

This is all a faith thing, God will perform only according to your faith. (Matthew 9 vs 29) Faith is seeing things the way God sees them and believing that God will do what He said He will do despite the circumstances. Without Faith it is impossible to please God. Faith is also a channel through which a human being taps into the power source of God. Faith without works is dead. Faith believes what God said no matter how unreasonable it may seem. Faith is the master key to your healing. Faith is reasoning with God about His Word and acting on it. So walk as much as possible in holiness so you don't give the devil permission to afflict you anyhow.

THROUGH APPLYING GODS WORD

Secondly, you must use the Word of God as your weapon against the devil. Jesus modeled this when he was tempted in the wilderness. Every time the devil suggested a temptation, Jesus countered by quoting scripture. He did not argue with the devil. He did not say "I am not hungry", but He simply quoted scripture from memory. We must do the same. The power is in God's Word and the devil fears it. Don't ever try to argue with the devil, he is better at arguing than you he has thousands of years of experience. You can't convince the devil with logic and your opinion, but you can use what makes him tremble – the truth of God. Memorizing scripture is absolutely essential to resisting the devil. Like Jesus the truth must be stored in your hearts, ready to be spoken. If you do not have any bible verses memorized you have no bullets in your gun!

- ✓ The Word is spirit and life (Jn 6:63, *"The Spirit gives life; the flesh counts for nothing. The words I have spoken to you are spirit and they are life."*)
- ✓ The Word of the Lord endures forever (1Pet. 1:25, *"but the word of the Lord stands for ever. And this is the word that was preached to you."*)
- ✓ The Word or the scriptures can not be broken (Jn 10:35b *"to whom the word of God came – and the scriptures cannot be broken"*)
- ✓ The Word of God does not return to Him void, it accomplishes that for which it has been sent. (Isaiah 55:11, *"so is my word that goes out from my mouth; it will not return to me empty, but will accomplish what I desire and achieve the purpose for which I sent it."*)
- ✓ The Word of God does not change (Ps 89:34, *"I will not violate my covenant or alter what my lips have uttered".*)

So what you need to do first of all is to look for the appropriate healing scriptures and meditate on them. Even if it is only one scripture it goes a long way. One scripture I love when it comes to healing is Romans 8: 11, *"And if the Spirit of him who raised Jesus from the dead is living in you, he who raised Christ from the dead will also give life to your mortal bodies through his Spirit who lives in you."* As you meditate on the Word your mind and your spirit man come into agreement and your miraculous healing takes place. Once the spirit man and the mind are in agreement the body automatically aligns itself to what they are saying.

4. **REMEMBER DIVINE HEALING IS YOUR PORTION**

We can't do it as the world does it, we may be in this world but we are not of this world, we are spirit and we share in the divinity of God. Therefore we walk in divine health and divine healing. Under normal circumstances when we are unwell we panic because the truth about Jesus being the healer has not been revealed to us by the Spirit of God. Ask God to reveal Himself to you as Jehovah Raphe.

Meditate on God's goodness and remember He will not put you to shame for whatever temptation you go through God has a way out for you *(2 Corinthians 10:13,14)*. All healing promises in the Word of God apply to all diseases including diseases like HIV/ AIDS, diabetes, hypertension, cancer etc. These so called incurable diseases are not special in the eyes of God; it is man who has made them so complicated. Be rest assured Jesus heals all diseases including HIV/AIDS, sugar disease, hypertension, cancer and so on, there is indeed nothing impossible for them that believe. It is really about believing because as a man thinks so is he! What are you thinking about yourself and your illness? Are you blaming yourself or condemning yourself? Stop! Forgive yourself and stop feeling guilty after all when you repent and ask God for forgiveness He forgives and forgets.

Due to the pain from some illness or the other, we are in such a vulnerable state so we are easily swayed into alternative methods of acquiring healing and health. It is very easy to convince any person who is in pain and does not know who they are in Christ because they are lacking maturity and faith to look for alternative forms of treatment even, witch craft. Such people will normally begin to convince themselves that God can answer their prayers in different ways and that it is okay for them to consult or seek medication from witch-doctors, and herbalists while they wait for God to heal them when in actual fact; He has already done it.

I want us to understand that for one reason or another we will get sick and have physical affliction. Whether sickness and disease come because of sin, infirmities, wrong spiritual foundations or just human error caused by not taking good care of our bodies we must remember that divine healing is our portion. Now when this happens we should in addition to repentance, deliverance and fasting also prayerfully seek medical attention. God created plants and herbs that contain medicinal properties and He has also given wisdom to individuals to develop remedies and procedures to relieve us from pain. This may not have been God's original plan for us but because we find ourselves in these circumstances by our own doing, God allows His permissive Will to provide supernatural healing through applied natural remedies and procedures. As we receive treatment in medical facilities it is very important that we remain in prayer focusing on God having faith that God will use the healthcare workers whom He created and gave wisdom to minister to us.

Because this afflictions make us so vulnerable we should ensure that we are not deceived into considering any other source of healing especially any that is spiritually inclined from witch doctors, fortune tellers or spiritualist. Any activities that include any form of ungodly meditation must be by all means avoided. My advice to you is to prayerfully seek a medical facility and take medication as prescribed while believing God for total healing and restoration. It has been proven through several research studies that patients who pray in addition to receiving medication heal faster and better than those who don't. Therefore, continue listening to recorded messages on healing, meditate on the Word of God, listen to Praise and Worship songs until your level of faith is lifted. Avoid thinking any negative thoughts about your condition, God is well able to heal you, after all your life is in His hands, you will not die but live to declare the works of the Lord. God's divine healing is permanent that is what every believer must desire.

CHAPTER FIVE

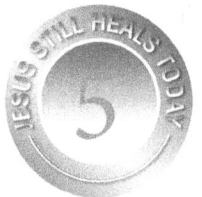

MAINTAINING YOUR HEALING

It is important to realize that the devil is tenacious and he will keep trying to bring back the sickness or disease. This is where you need to continuously resist the devil as in James 4:7-8 which says, "Submit yourselves then to God. Resist the devil, and he will flee from you". Try by all means to accommodate only positive thoughts. Each time you have a negative thought, replace it with a positive one.

Be conversant with what the Word of God says about your health and believe it as true. Trust in the Lord with all your heart, lean not on your own understanding no matter how much the devil tries to bring negative thoughts. Confess the Word of God loudly as often as you can. Affirm your healing and divine health. Do not be ignorant of God's promises for health.

Most importantly, be holy as God is holy. To be holy is to be separated from sin or impurity and set apart for a special purpose. Separation and purity are the core of holiness. Thus Jesus is said to be holy (Mk 1:24, 1 Peter 2: 21-22). Therefore we need to watch and pray so we do not enter into temptation: the spirit is willing but the flesh is weak. Matt. 26:41. A call to sainthood is a call to holiness. For God has not called us unto uncleanness, but unto holiness (1 Thess 4:7). Look at what a few of the scriptures say on the issue of holiness;

In Psalm 91:1 dwelling in the shelter of the Most High God, assures us of rest in the shadow of the Almighty. Now what does it take to dwell in the shelter of the Most High God? It obviously takes holiness. You cannot enter the presence of God with sin or blemish!

In Deuteronomy 28 we read of the results of obedience and of disobedience. In Leviticus 26: 3-13 we also read of the reward of obedience. So we actually get rewarded for living this holy life.

Holiness is basically a choice we make, as in Deuteronomy 30: 15-16. If you chose to be holy and fulfil your part of the covenant that you made with God the day you got saved, then you will obviously receive the rewards that He has promised you such as prosperity, divine health, protection, long life etc…

In John 15:7 Jesus tells us that if we remain in Him and His words remain in us, we can ask Him anything and He will do it. Look at verse 10, there He is telling us what it takes to remain in Him, He says, "If you obey my commands you will remain in me…" and in verse 17 He gives us His command as "Love each other". Love is the opposite of sin, so in other words He was saying, "Do not sin." Obviously if you really love someone you would not like to see them hurt, so you will not lie to them, you will not backbite them, you will not gossip about them, you will be loyal and faithful to your spouse, you will not steal from the one you love, etc..

Living a holy life is so serious that if we regard sin in our hearts God will not hear us, Psalm 66:18. You may have been praying for something for a long time, just check and see if there is unconfessed sin in your life, maybe God can't hear you. In 2 Corinthians 6:17-18 and 7:1 Paul reminds us of the promises given us in our covenant with the Lord. Paul is saying here that since God has promised us all these lovely things, why can't we just be holy so we can receive the blessings set before us? Is it too much to ask?

Galatians 5: 16-26 is very clear; we need to live by the spirit so that we do not gratify the sinful nature. Those of us who live in sin will not inherit the Kingdom of God! The Kingdom of God is the abundant life that has been promised us through out the Word of God. God is not so interested in the fact that we will be going to heaven when we die, He is more interested in us experiencing Heaven here on earth! He sent the Holy Spirit to come and change our characters so that we can become more and more Christ like ensuring our access to the wonderful promises of God.

In John 17:11 Jesus is praying for us to God, asking God to protect us by the power of His name, so that we may be **one** as they are **one.** Jesus here is saying that we need to be in agreement *Spirit, Soul and Body* as God the Father, the Son and the Holy Spirit are in agreement. Now for us to be in agreement Spirit, Soul and Body we need to be holy, if the Spirit, Soul and Body are not in agreement then we are in sin. SIN therefore can be defined as; the state in which the Spirit, Soul and Body are not in agreement. So for us to be one as the Trinity is one, we need to have no sin in our lives!

As long as we walk in holiness we will resist the devil and he will flee from us (James 4:7b). You see the devil is so afraid of holiness, if you have no sin in you he has no permission or opportunity to afflict you. When you walk in holiness, indeed no weapon formed against you shall prosper. Once you fall into sin he has permission to afflict you immediately, it is like the protective shield around you disappears. Remember the devil prowls around as a roaring lion seeking whom to devour (1Peter:8), while he is seeking whom to devour and he finds you with sin he pounces on you. So remain holy and the devil will have no reason to touch you or yours. When the devil afflicts you he is only coming to get what belongs to him, sin.

Let us rid ourselves of all malice and deceit, hypocrisy, envy and slander of every kind (1 Peter 2:1), let us be built into a spiritual house to be a holy priesthood, offering spiritual sacrifices acceptable to God through Jesus Christ (1 Peter 2:5).

Therefore, first of all we need to make a decision to consciously avoid sin, and then secondly, ask God to deliver us from evil. This is the part of the Lord's prayer that we often omit. We need to ask for the grace to overcome temptation to sin, God is faithful enough to give us the grace and as we continue like this eventually we will live a blameless life without much effort, it will become our life style.

Lastly, we need to live in constant repentance, especially now as we begin this walk into holiness, we need to be in constant repentance like David. You see despite his shortfalls, David was the apple of God's eye, because he knew how to go to God and repent each time he sinned (Psalm 51).

In conclusion we need to take the following steps:
1. Repent of all known and unknown sin.
2. Make a decision to consciously resist sin in which ever form it comes (Colossians 3:1-17) .
3. Ask the Holy Spirit to deliver us from evil and give us the grace to overcome temptation.
4. Walk in constant repentance being conscious of sin.

CHAPTER SIX

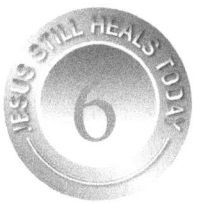

EPILOGUE – WITH GOD ALL THINGS ARE POSSIBILE

In this chapter I would like to testify of the healing power of God over my own life. I am a living testimony of the fact that God heals all diseases. In my life I have been afflicted on several occasions with sickness and disease. Since I was a little baby, just after my birth I was attacked with whooping cough. By the grace of God I survived though my cousin who was slightly older than me in the same house died of whooping cough. Thereafter, according to my step-fathers testimony I was a sickly child and it is a miracle that I survived to this age.

So far I can give testimony to over 10 surgical procedures carried out on my body. As far back as 1982 I remember I had an acute appendicitis while on a train in Germany where I was studying. I really don't know what happened but when I woke up I found myself in a hospital bed. The train had to make an emergency stop in a small town and I was transported by ambulance to a hospital where the emergency laparotomy was performed. This was going to be the beginning of the many surgical procedures. During this time I was not born again and I did not know God as my personal savior so I will lie if I say I prayed. Latter during the 12 years I spent in Germany I underwent surgery on my wrists because of ganglions.

In January 1997 I came to know the Lord and I quickly began to study the word of God. I came to realize that Jesus had done it all at the cross, but despite this knowledge I continued to be afflicted by sickness and disease. I cannot talk about all the incidences but I will narrate just a few. In 2004, I suffered a severe abdominal pain that started with a tooth extraction. After my tooth was extracted, I had severe pain so the doctor ordered that I receive diclofenac injections three times daily. By the time I was to receive my sixth injection one evening I started to throw up and I had a very severe abdominal pain. I was rushed to the hospital but unfortunately there was no surgeon to rule out any intestinal obstruction or perforation. I had never experienced so much pain in my life, even child birth was nothing compared to this pain. If people could die of pain, I should have died that night. Anyway to cut a long story short, the next day I was diagnosed with a perforated large intestine and was immediately sent to theatre for a laparotomy. This was a very big scar from the top of my abdomen in the epigastric region to right down about 10 cm below my umbilicus.

Okay the operation was successful and I was alive. I was not allowed to eat any solids and was on a drip. After about 14 days I began to have temperatures and I was vomiting since again. The doctor examined me and thought I must have an intestinal obstruction, so I had to go to theatre again. Now you must realize that at this point I had lost a lot of weight and I was what we call 'wasted'. Form the physical point of view there was no way I could have survived another operation, so I resisted at first. But with the pain and the continued vomiting I had to give in. At this point I was so sure that I would not survive the operation. So I decided to prepare myself spiritually and it was then that God sent a nurse to pray with me. This lady had just been recruited for part-time and she also agreed with me later that it was so divine. While by the grace of God I pulled through though I must say here that everyone else had given up hope except my husband who believed I would pull through. This was a miracle from the throne room of Jehovah God Himself. I have healed completely and have never experienced any abdominal problems as a result of the operation, it's like the scar is the only reminder of what God can do.

Another such event happened in the recent past, July 2014. I had been suffering from what we call "herniated lumbar disc" for about 6 months and in July I went through spinal surgery to correct it so that I could be relieved of the pain. Once again the operation went well, but after about 3 weeks the wound opened and became septic. So I was admitted again for cleaning and secondary suture. This was a very painful experience; if you were there while they were cleaning the wound you would have felt sorry for me. I cried and screamed like a little child. This went on for about 10 days and finally when the wound was clean enough it was sutured and closed. Today am totally healed I have no pain whatsoever, if you see the scar you won't believe that was the same deep open wound that was there. Those that were there with me can bear witness. God once again did a miracle.

During both these events I took time to talk to God. In both cases when I was at my worst I asked God to cut short my life. I was in so much pain and I preferred to go home to the Father instead of living such a useless life of pain and sorrow. God did not allow this to happen, He made me realize that the purposes for which He created me are still not fully accomplished. I appreciate now more than ever that God is the one who determines when I depart this earthly body. It is clear that once you are a child of God, God takes charge and it does not matter what the enemy brings your way you will not die but see the goodness of the Lord in the land of the living. God heals all diseases and for as long as your assignment here on earth is not finished you will not die.

During another episode of illness, I was so sick that I had actually experienced myself coming out of my body. I was sleeping on our matrimony bed and I felt myself falling deep down into a tunnel at a very fast speed. While I was going down I saw the words of these scriptures flying in front of me; "Greater is He who is within me than he who is in the world; I will not die but live to see the salvation of the Lord; I will see the goodness of the Lord in the land of the living". Suddenly after these words had flown in front of me, I woke up and got healed miraculously. I could eat without vomiting and my temperature had gone down. Once again I saw the hand of God.

There are so many other testimonies and experiences including some of my family members and my patients that prove to me that God does heal all diseases and that Jesus still heals us today. Have faith in God and you shall be healed.

CHAPTER SEVEN

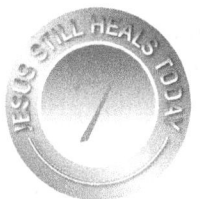

HEALING SCRIPTURES AND AFFIRMATIONS

Physical Healing Scriptures - All Bible references are from The Amplified Bible

Most people believe that God is Able to heal but they aren't sure whether He will heal them. I encourage you to carefully read each of these scriptures. Notice how much God wants to heal you. You don't have to do something to earn His love or His healing touch just believe what God says and do what He tells you to do.

Start by speaking these verses out loud. Meditate on them. Believe them. Speak His Word and trust His ability and His willingness to heal all of your diseases.

Psalm 118:17
I shall not die but live, and shall declare the works and recount the illustrious acts of the Lord.

Psalm 147:3
He heals the brokenhearted and binds up their wounds [curing

their pains and their sorrows].

Psalm 103:1-3
BLESS (AFFECTIONATELY, gratefully praise) the Lord, O my soul; and all that is [deepest] within me, bless His holy name!

Bless (affectionately, gratefully praise) the Lord, O my soul, and forget not [one of] all His benefits, who forgives [every one of] all your iniquities, who heals [each one of] all your diseases.

Proverbs 4:20-22
My son, attend to my words; consent and submit to my sayings. Let them not depart from your sight; keep them in the center of your heart. For they are life to those who find them, healing and health to all their flesh.

Exodus 23:25
You shall serve the Lord your God; He shall bless your bread and water, and will take sickness from your midst.

Jeremiah 17:14
Heal me, O Lord, and I shall be healed; save me, and I shall be saved, for you are my praise.

Proverbs 3:7-8
Be not wise in your own eyes; reverently fear and worship the Lord and turn [entirely] away from evil. It shall be health to your nerves and sinews, and marrow and moistening to your bones.

3 John 1:2
Beloved, I pray that you may prosper in every way and [that your body] may keep well, even as [I know] your soul keeps well and prospers.

Mark 16:17-18
And these attesting signs will accompany those who believe: in my name they will drive out demons; they will speak in new languages;

they will pick up serpents; and [even] if they drink anything deadly, it will not hurt them; they will lay their hands on the sick, and they will get well.

Matthew 9:20-22

And behold, a woman who had suffered from a flow of blood for twelve years came up behind Him and touched the fringe of His garment; for she kept saying to herself, If I only touch His garment, I shall be restored to health. Jesus turned around and, seeing her, He said, Take courage, daughter! Your faith has made you well. And at once the woman was restored to health.

Matthew 4:23-24

And He went about all Galilee, teaching in their synagogues and preaching the good news (Gospel) of the kingdom, and healing every disease and every weakness and infirmity among the people. So the report of Him spread throughout all Syria, and they brought Him all who were sick, those afflicted with various diseases and torments, those under the power of demons, and epileptics, and paralyzed people, and He healed them.

Matthew 8:16-17

When evening came, they brought to Him many who were under the power of demons, and He drove out the spirits with a word and restored to health all who were sick. And thus He fulfilled what was spoken by the prophet Isaiah, He Himself took [in order to carry away] our weaknesses and infirmities and bore away our diseases.

James 5:14-15

Is anyone among you sick? He should call in the church elders (the spiritual guides). And they should pray over him, anointing him with oil in the Lord's name. And the prayer [that is] of faith will save him who is sick, and the Lord will restore him; and if he has committed sins, he will be forgiven.

Confessions for physical healing:

"I know that it's God's will for me to be healthy and whole. I Praise the Lord and thank Him for healing all of my diseases as I put my faith and trust in Him."

Father God, I thank you for creating me in your image. I praise you that I am fearfully and wonderfully made. I confess that you are the God that heals, my Great Physician. I thank you for healing my body from the top of my head to the soles of my feet. I thank you for regenerating every bone, joint, tendon, ligament, tissue, organ, and blood cell of my body. This is the day that the Lord has made; I will rejoice and be glad in it.
AMEN.

Steps to deliverance from the spirit of disease and infirmity

1. Repentance and rededication to Christ
2. Take authority of the infection and command the spirit of infirmity to leave to body
3. Command restoration of the immune system
4. Command all organs in the body to be healed and restored
5. Give thanks to God for healing and restoration